I0440494

Healthy Lifestyle Report:

Fat-Burning and Motivational Tips

Proven Tips You Can Use

To

Burn Fat, Lose Weight and Stay Motivated

RON KNESS

Contents

Introduction

B e honest: When you look in a mirror, which bit do you hate the most? Is it those 'Love Handles' that have sprouted up? Does your tummy wobble a little too much now? Or do you wear baggy clothes that cover a multitude of sins?

Not everyone builds up fat in the same area on the body but if you are like most people with this problem, you will want the same result - you want it to disappear!

This excess fat goes on so easy, so why does it require so much effort to make it come off again? Everyone talks about the latest fat burning supplement or 'super' food but it is hard to determine what is a gimmick and what really works. Is it possible to burn more fat?

You are told that to lose weight you need to lose the fat stores from around your body. Most people know the general way you get energy from your body is from the food we eat but without knowing how the body uses the different food groups to do so.

You want to make your body use fat for energy, which makes sense if you want to lose weight, but without knowing how your body makes and burns fat, trying to increase the amount of fat your body actually consuming is like trying to figure out the latest technical appliance without the manual. It would be just guess work with no real results.

In this report we are going to show you some proven ways to get rid of fat, thereby losing weight, along with some motivational tips to help you stay the course during your weight loss journey.

10 Instant Fat-Burning Tips to Give You the Body You've Always Wanted

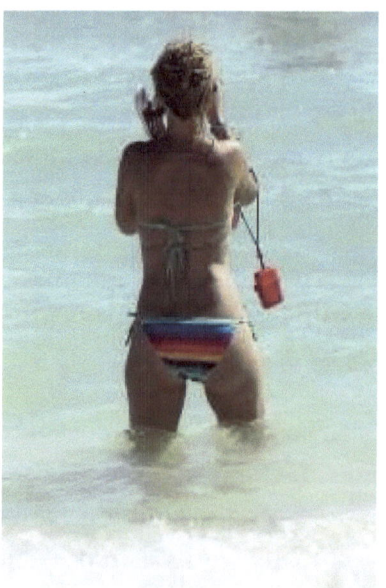

Most of your body's daily energy is fueled by the breakdown of fat and carbohydrates (carbs), but during and after exercise your body will use protein for both energy and to repair the muscles. However, the amount of fat and carbs used by your body varies depending on what type of work or exercise you are doing. Sometimes your body uses more fat than carbs to fuel your daily activities, and other times it will use more carbs than fat. So are there any benefits, in terms of weight loss, of doing high intensity exercise over low intensity exercise?

When you are doing aerobic high intensity exercises, for instance cycling very fast, running hard your body needs to access fuel fast and get it processed into a form your cells can use, and the quickest way for your body to do that is to break down carbs.

Because it takes longer to access and process stored body fat, if your body needs energy fast, it turns to carbs first for fuel and uses a lower amount of body fat.

If, on the other hand, you are doing an exercise activity that is less

intensive, for instance walking at a moderate pace or leisurely cycling, your body can take longer to access fuel and it uses your body fat more than carbs for this energy. But less intensive activities burn 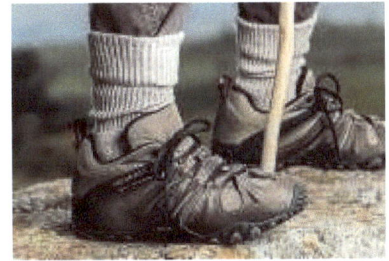 far less calories and you need to do them for much longer in order to burn the same amount of calories as the higher intensity version.

Take, for example, cycling. If you were to ride a bike at a leisurely pace, at less than 10 miles per hour, you would burn around 280 calories per hour. If you were to then ride the same bike quite

energetically at around 15 miles per hour, your calorie use would jump up to around 590 calories per hour, so you would only need to exercise for 30 minutes in order to burn 280 calories. Even though your body uses a lower percentage 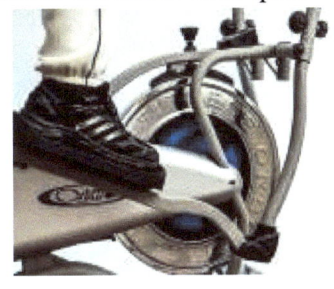 of fat overall when exercising at high intensity, you still probably end up burning off more fat by exercising at a high intensity than you would by doing an hour of low intensity exercise.

But regardless of what type of exercise you do, the most important principle for weight loss is to use up more calories per day than you take into your body.

That doesn't mean starving yourself by taking in only 200-300 calories and then spending 3 hours a day at the gym.

Not only would that be extremely unhealthy and something that you would not be able to sustain for long, but not eating enough could cause your body to begin breaking down muscles to use for energy instead.

Everyone needs to take in a minimum amount of energy from food in order just to keep your body ticking over. Everything your body does requires energy - breathing, pumping blood around your body, even things like sitting, watching TV and sleeping. Depending on your height and weight, a normally active lifestyle can require anything from 1500 - 3000 calories per day just to do day-to-day activities. The trick to losing weight is to know how much energy you are taking in and then make sure you are using up 500-600 calories of energy MORE than   you take in. Doing that on a daily basis will see you begin to lose one pound per week – 52 pounds in just one year.

Many people don't know where to begin but you've come to the right place. Here are 10 tips that you can put in place right now to help you on your way to a healthier life and to start burning off that excess weight...

Eat Regularly

If you regularly skip meals, or have very long periods of time between meals, rather than lose weight you will actually force your body to start holding on to the food energy you have taken in, and over time that can actually lead to your body storing more fat not less. Eating a minimum of 3 meals and some healthy snacks in-between will keep your metabolism higher.

Less and More

While you should definitely aim to eat at least 3 times per day, having to process and digest large intakes of calories can hinder your body's metabolism and give you peaks and dips in your blood sugar. It is much better to spread your intake out over the day, eating 4 - 6 smaller meals and keep the calories down to around 300 - 350 calories per meal. Try not to eat too much processed food or food with a high sugar content (such as cakes, sweets, sugary drinks).

Instead make sure you have plenty of natural choices, including vegetables and fresh fruits, for a good healthy lifestyle.

Say YES to Breakfast

A common misconception is that if you don't eat breakfast you will eat less throughout the day and so lose weight. That is not very sensible thinking at all.

Breakfast is important to wake the body out of sleep mode and it kick starts your daily metabolism. Rather than making you eat more, a healthy breakfast will make it less likely that you will have to snack on something mid-morning, especially if you eat a slow-release carbohydrate like oats. Rather than overload your bloodstream with a huge hit of sugar, slow-release carbohydrates (sometimes called complex or

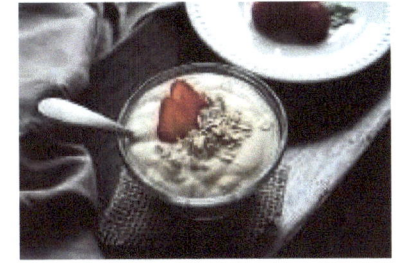

good carbs) release a steady stream of energy. This is much better for you as you don't get the massive peak then drop in blood sugar which sends your body a message that you need to take in (eat) more fuel, so preventing you from eating calories you don't really need.

Good Carb, Bad Carb

You may think a carb is a carb and they were all created equal, but nothing could be further from the truth.

The term 'carbohydrate' applies to any organic plant compound that can be broken down by the body into sugars that the body can then use for energy, but carbohydrates themselves come in many forms. So why are some better than others?

It depends on how quickly the body is able to break them down and how fast the resulting sugars enter into the blood stream. A good carbohydrate is one that takes the body both time and energy to break it down into a useable energy source; things like lentils and beans, whole grains (like oats, brown rice) and vegetables. A bad carbohydrate is one that takes the body no time to at all to process, and because of that all the energy released from that carbohydrate rushes into the bloodstream, causing a massive spike in blood sugar. Once that spike has gone, the resulting rapid dip in blood sugar levels can give us the craving to eat again.

Bad carbohydrates are usually found in processed or refined foods - things like sugary drinks, cakes and cookies, chocolate or candy - and take very little digesting. A can of fizzy sugary drink can enter the bloodstream within 20 SECONDS!

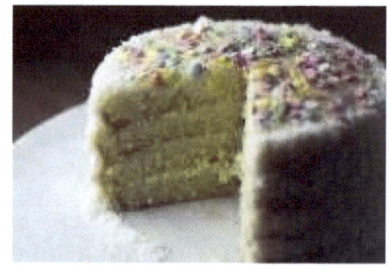

So by replacing these types of food with a slow-release food, not only will you be fuller for longer but your body is much less likely to store the excess energy as fat.

What the Eye Doesn't See …

Studies have shown that our perception of food is based a lot on what we see. Diners may not have noticed it, but the size of the average dinner plate used in the home has jumped from 9" in diameter up to 12".

That may not seem like much of an increase until you realize that is a 40% increase in the surface area, so that's 40% MORE food we expect to see on our plate at every meal. So if we are using a large plate for our meals, but don't fill it, then we feel that we haven't had all the food we should have and we go looking for more.

This is one of the easiest solutions to put into practice... simply swap your 12" plate back down to a smaller one. Psychologically your brain will tell you that your plate is full, and you won't be tempted into putting that extra food on your plate as there simply won't be any room. We can all be guilty of not noticing what we eat. Even at mealtimes, we can hurry through our food and it's only after we develop a bloated or bulging feeling do we realize we have overeaten. This can happen because we haven't given our brain the chance to catch up to the amount of food we are eating. By the time the brain can register we have eaten enough, it's too late.

Instead of rushing, take time to enjoy every mouthful of food you eat. By thoroughly chewing each mouthful of food, you not only give your brain time to send out the 'You're Full' sign, but you are helping to begin breaking down your food.

How many ordinary restaurants put the calorie count of their dishes on the menu? Would it come as a surprise to learn that the meals you eat in a restaurant can contain over TWICE the calories of the same meal you would cook at home?

Eating out can be a big potential pitfall for putting on weight. It is harder to appreciate how much food you are actually eating. You tend not to register little nibbles like bread, butter, breadsticks, canapes, cocktails, etc.

The temptation is there to have 3 or 4 courses because someone else is doing the cooking: or 'it all looks so nice': Some dishes come laden with hidden additional calories in rich sauces and garnishes.

If you have a tendency towards eating out regularly, try to have more home-cooked meals where you can control fully what healthy food is going into your meals and so keep a check on your calorie intake.

Alcohol – The Calorie Ninja

Drinking alcohol is probably one of the biggest areas of self-denial people can have. Because it comes in a glass, it is seen as harmless. But gram for gram, alcohol has almost as many calories as fat!

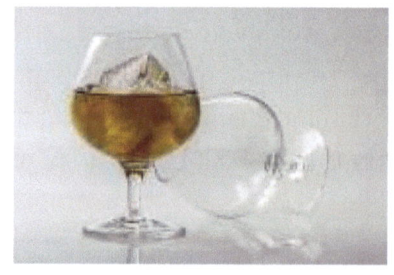

And when you are drinking alcohol, it stops your body from burning fat as the alcohol calories are used up first.

The calories in alcohol have no nutritional value for the body so they are 'empty' calories, but as they are used first. the body will store the extra calories from your food as fat. But how bad can they be?

Beer contains 180 calories per pint (approx. 500 ml). Wine, which you would think would be better because you drink it in smaller amounts, contains 85 calories in a small 125 ml glass. Not too bad you think? Well compared to beer, that is 340 calories per 500 ml.

That is almost double!

In an average bottle of wine, there are around 500 calories. What about spirits – the smaller the better right? Spirts, on average, have about 75 calories in a 35ml shot. Which is a massive 1035 calories per 500ml. When you add in the mixer, it pushes it over 100 calories per small drink.

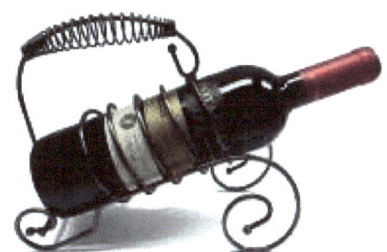

Two drinks per day is enough to add 1pound of weight or more per week. Recognizing the amount of extra calories, you could be taking in through alcohol, as well as the other effects of increasing your appetite and stopping fat from burning within your body, should motivate you to try and cut down on the amount you are drinking.

Don't Swap One Bad Habit for Another

Changing over from drinking alcohol to soft drinks can be helpful in reducing calories, but they need to be the right kind of drink. Soda, fruit juice, and cordials may on the surface seem like a better choice, but there are hidden dangers in these too from excess sugar.

In a regular 330ml can of sugary soft drink, there is 40g of sugar, which is 139 calories. Even fruit juice, can contain really high amounts of sugar, pushing the calorie count up.

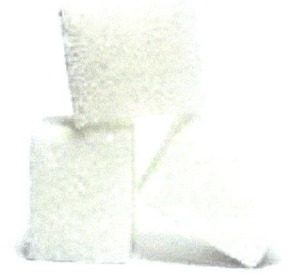

It might seem a fair swap, but drinking just one can per day will amount to 50,735 calories in a year.

In terms of weight gain, that is 25 pounds!

Without doing anything else, changing over from a sugary soft drink over to a diet version will help you lose 14 of those 25 pounds you gained. From strictly a calorie standpoint, not a bad exchange for 1 can of soft drink! However there are other things at play with diet soda that are not good for you either, like the caramel coloring and artificial sweeteners.

If the math is not working for you here is why. It takes 2,000 excess calories to gain a pound, but requires burning 3,500 calories to lose that pound. Fair? No. Reality? Yes! That is one reason why it is so much easier to gain weight than to lose it.

Water, Water Everywhere

When it comes to liquids, nothing does your body as much good as cool refreshing water. It hydrates the muscles to help them work more efficiently, it helps the blood and organs filter toxins out of the body, and surprisingly drinking water stops your body from retaining water. Added to that, there are no calories or harmful chemical additives in water.

If you find yourself craving something to eat, but aren't sure what it is you want, try drinking a glass or two of water first. We can get signals mixed up in out body and we can feel hungry when really we are just thirsty.

Tea for Good Health

The properties of green tea have been known for a while, but studies have confirmed that if you drink tea, and green tea in particular, it will increase your metabolism even when you are resting. More than that, it can also help release stored body fat.

Rather than drink the ready-made, pre-packaged versions, put the kettle on and take time to brew up your own.

That way you can steer clear of any nasty hidden extras, like sugar.

Time to Get Moving

Careful eating is not going to be enough to give you the healthy lifestyle you want. To burn off that excess body fat, you are going to need to begin exercising sooner rather than later. But we are not talking about running a marathon or spending 5 hours a day in the gym.

You can make great strides by doing 30 minutes of exercise every day, whether that is walking, swimming, cycling or anything else that requires effort, so things like house work, gardening, playing with the children and anything else that raises your heart rate and makes you sweat a little.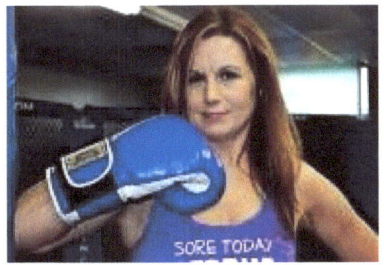
You can even break it down into smaller 10 minute bursts. They all add up to burning more calories.

The key to making exercise a useful part of your weight loss routine is regularity. You must keep up your exercise daily, and it will be made much easier and more enjoyable if you find something that you really like doing. Add variety in the kind of activity you do. Don't just stick to walking or swimming - try to add in some free weights or a little resistance band training.

If you have not exercised for a long time, or perhaps have health issues, there is no need to despair. There are exercise programs available for all levels of fitness and ability.

Take a look online to see what guidelines and training is recommended for your situation, as well as speaking to your health practitioner for practical help.

Success of failure lies in your hands. No-one else can burn that fat for you, but if you apply and follow through on these tips, you will see results. Each one of these tips is proven to bring results, and the more of these tips you can put into practice in your life, the greater the results you will see. Even if you can't put all of the tips into practice, don't let that deter you from using the others on your way to a longer, healthier lifestyle.

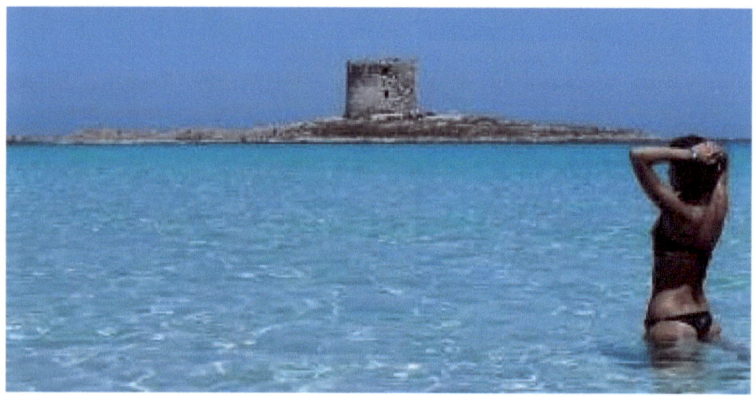

16 Motivational Tips to Help You Lose Weight

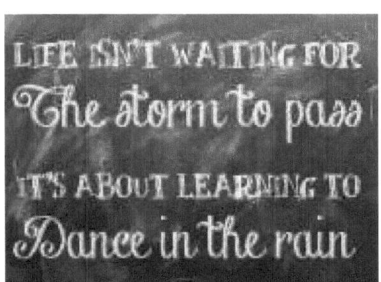

D o you remember how excited you felt when you first decided you were going to lose weight and start making all new healthy lifestyle choices? You were so enthusiastic and full of hope. You flung open your cupboards and began your healthy lifestyle spring cleaning … OUT went all the chocolate cookies and fat-loaded snacks. OUT went the ice cream in your freezer. You even kicked your secret stash of chocolates into the trash.

You were a food-shopping genius, filled with steely determination that nothing in the aisles of your supermarket would ever tempt you to allow those calorie-laden, sugar traps to enter the temple that was your body.

Your determination took you through the horrors of the office birthday party without a crumb of cake passing your lips, as you pictured yourself in that fantastic new outfit you passed in the shop window last week.

But then, something terrible happens...you hit the dieting equivalent of the runner's wall. Suddenly, it's not all sunshine and roses. You're only a few weeks into your new lifestyle choice, and it's beginning to feel a whole lot harder. It's no longer fun and exciting. Your motivation takes a beating because you weren't expecting it to be this tough. You start thinking that after these weeks of deprivation and denial, almost all that excess 90lb should be gone, shouldn't it? And yet you still have another 78lb to go.

Your initial weight loss has slowed down to a trickle, so you begin to lose confidence in what you are doing. Then you look at your meals -you're bored with the repetitive round of dull steamed vegetables and grilled skinless chicken, night after night.

One cold, wet, rainy night you arrive home soaked to the skin, freezing cold and starving. Opening the fridge door, you see your 'delicious' salad and it leaves you dejected and miserable. Your mind and body start a revolution…'HOT food' they chant in your head...'Hot Food. Tasty Food. Hot food, Tasty Food' and you start to believe it.

You might put up a little struggle, just for show to make yourself feel better about what you are about to do, but finally you relent and give in. As you sink your teeth into a steaming hot pie that fell out of the fridge into the microwave, you tell yourself it can't hurt having it 'just this once'.

But the next day, you think to yourself that you'll start again on Monday when you feel better, but how many times have you said that? Truthfully ask yourself… did you every start again when Monday came around? And then the vicious circle starts again a few months later.

Many things can make you want to go off the healthy lifestyle rails - ill health, a bad day at work, financial troubles to name just a few. But everyone gets bad days in life. So why is it that only some people, after they have had a few slip-ups, end up losing their motivation and giving up? After all, it leaves them feeling bad about themselves, and nobody likes to feel like that.

We all know getting fit and losing weight isn't easy. That in itself is enough to put some people off trying and encourages others to think that they are doomed to fail, so why bother to try and keep going when the going gets tough?

What Needs to Change?

GOAL SETTING

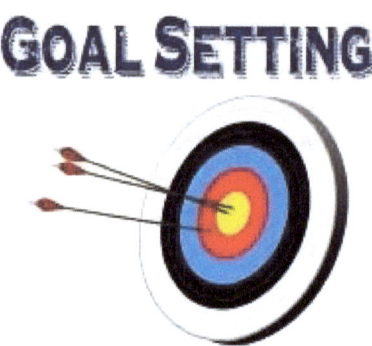

L et's go back to the beginning. What is the difference between the time that you first made the decision to improve your lifestyle and the decision to stop? Wasn't it the way you felt and thought about things? You had weighted up the pros and cons of your life at that moment and knew that you had to change things inside your body to be a healthier individual. You looked ahead to the benefits you would gain by improving your lifestyle and that gave you the motivation to want to succeed.

It has been shown that the key to losing weight and keeping it off is your attitude. Your positive desire for success, not just in losing weight but in maintaining a healthy lifestyle long term, is more important than how much exercise you do or how many calories you eat. It is this desire that drives and motivates you to carry on. You need to keep this motivation fresh and it does need topping up occasionally. As we said, everybody has good AND bad days, but if you deal with each bad day in a positive way, you can minimize the impact each one has on your life.

If you have found yourself repeating this cycle of dropping and regaining weight more times than you care to think about, then it's time to readjust the way you look at things. Start by adopting a realistic view of what you are about to do. Achieving a lasting weight loss is a slow process and it is so easy to become dejected and give up before you reach your goal.

If you can relate to the scenario above and feel your motivation is starting to wane, then these motivation tips will keep you and your quest for a healthy lifestyle choice to lose weight and eat healthily on the winning track.

Here are some great motivational ways to help if you are losing steam but not pounds:

Set Small Achievable Goals

When you are ready to start, it's really important that you don't set yourself up to fail. You may have a really positive attitude and are determined, but more is needed than that. Starting a new healthier lifestyle implies you have an end goal - somewhere you ultimately want to end up. HOW you plan to get to that end goal goes a long way in ensuring whether you succeed or fail.

Imagine yourself in this situation: You are standing at the bottom of a really high mountain. You look up but can't see the top of it as it disappears up into the clouds. Then you are told that you have to walk all the way up to the very top. The size of the mountain in front of you makes you feel very small indeed but you set off walking up the mountain path. You walk for hours. Exhausted, you stop to see your progress but when you look back, you haven't come very far and still have a very long way to go. How much further would you go before you were dejected and decided to chuck it in and head back?

But what if, when you were about to set off, you were shown a little tent about 500 feet up the mountain and told that was where you needed to get to? Yes, it still takes effort to get there but you have something to focus on, something totally achievable to you. When you get there, you feel so much better at having finished the first stage. The next day, you are shown another tent 500 feet further up the mountain and you make your way there. How much further do you think you would get up that mountain? It might take a little longer to reach the top than trying to get there in one massive sustained effort, but it is much less likely you will be overwhelmed or worn down by the size of the task ahead of you.

That example demonstrates how, even with the best will in the world, the way we look at a task we have to achieve can have a massive effect on whether we ultimately succeed or fail.

So vowing to have to have perfect beach holiday for next summer is all well and good, but you need to examine the scale of what you are trying to accomplish. Deciding to lose 50 pounds in two months is completely unreasonable, especially if you want to keep losing weight in the same high amounts month in month out, but losing 10 pounds in two months is completely within your grasp. Your self-belief and confidence in your ability will get a huge boost, which will, in turn, encourage you to keep going. By setting and reaching more modest, achievable goals, you reinforce your determination to reach your target weight the more goals you reach.

If you have more than 20 or 30 pounds to lose, you need to take a hard look at the timescale you have given yourself to accomplish it and ask if it is reasonable and achievable long term. Trying to achieve too much in too little time is more likely to actually set you back, if not sabotage your efforts completely.

Think About Feeling Great and Not About the Weight Loss

Most people only change their food choices once they have decided to lose some weight. But what happens AFTER you lose weight? Because you aren't changing the basic way you think about food, once you reach your goal you go back to your old habits. This can lead to you to put back on all of the weight you have lost and that will discourage you from ever trying again.

You have to eat everyday so change your thinking from the negative 'I'm on a diet' to the much more positive and motivating 'This is a great healthy way of life'. By making healthy eating part of your lifestyle you not only feel better but you lose the weight... and keep it off.

Keeping a food journal can help build up your confidence and give you motivation to reach your goals

Have an Accountability Partner

It's easy to become discouraged so focus on what is going right. I know you're thinking to yourself ... 'If only I had the time and money to afford a personal trainer every day. That would make the job so much easier!' Not everybody can afford to do that, but it has been shown that the additional support of another person who is trying to achieve the same thing as you does help to keep you motivated and on track. So why not find a friend or join a group to help inspire you when you miss a workout or feel like giving up.

There is evidence that proves that people are much more likely to lose weight and keep it off if they are part of a group than those who don't.

Don't Ban Your Favorite Foods

Don't ban the food you love because it will just make you crave them even more. You can't eat THAT! What does that make you want to do? Don't you imagine how good it tastes?

You are depriving yourself of that fantastic food, because there will never ever be another pizza made ever again! Or, the world will run out of cocoa beans before 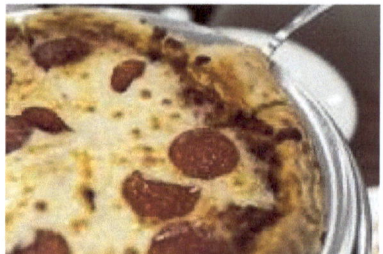 you ever have another chocolate! You know how ridiculous that sounds when you say it out loud but if you ban yourself from eating any of your most loved foods, all it will do is make you crave them even more.

It is better to limit and not eliminate less healthy choices. You are not trying to take all the joy out of your life because that would leave you in a very negative frame of mind. By allow yourself to have them in moderation, you will have a much more balanced attitude toward the food you eat. By having these food types, but less often, you will not feel like you are missing out on anything. It will make your determination to lose weight and stick to your goals much easier.

Pace Yourself

We know that when the excitement of imagining the 'new you' takes hold, you are over eager to make all of the changes at once, but the strain of trying to accomplish everything together is a recipe for disaster. These are bold new lifestyle changes you are putting in place - a brand new exercise program and a complete change in the way you think about and approach food, which can seem like a strict eating regime to begin with. It's no good trying to run a marathon if you can't walk 100 yards yet.

Remember your goal and that the best way to reach it is by making lots of small achievable steps. not huge over-reaching strides. So instead of making bold lifestyle changes that you are not exactly looking forward to and will not be able to stick to. decide instead to take realistic bite-sized action steps.

You Will Slip Up Now and Then. Get Over It!

It's the morning after the night before, and you wake to see the remains of a chunk of cake staring accusingly at you from the kitchen bench. You could swear you see the word FAIL spelled out in crumbs. Dejected, you want to reach for another slice because now you have undone all your hard work in a moment of madness and you can't face starting all over again.

Well guess what? You're human! Why does that surprise you? You may have slipped up and had a moment of weakness but we all do. Nobody is perfect and you're going to have to come to terms with the fact that it's okay to slip up now and again as long as you don't

let it get your down and discourage you from continuing. After all, how much damage can you have done? You need to eat 2,000 calories MORE than you use up in order to put l pound of fat on. So 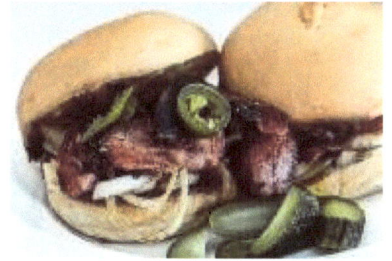 unless you ate an entire 3-tier wedding cake and washed it down with four cans of sugary drinks, I think you can safely say you haven't undone all your hard work.

BUT...if you do slip up, DON'T beat yourself up over it. Get the right perspective on what has happened - it was one slip up, not an avalanche! Then, use any ounce of motivation that you have in you to get yourself back on track. If you 'cheated' last night get over it and don't make it an excuse to have a Danish pastry for breakfast.

Simply tell yourself that today is a new day and recommit to your goal and make up for it.

Focus on What is Going Right

Everyone's emotions fluctuate. The pressures of life, problems and stresses can take their toll on anyone and sometimes we slip into a more negative frame of mind. Feeling like that makes it much easier to become discouraged because we have missed a workout or two or slipped up on our healthy eating.

To help raise yourself out of this way of thinking, stop focusing on what you haven't done, and start looking at what you HAVE accomplished. Take a few minutes to pat yourself on the back for all the good actions you have taken and all the goals you have reached so far. Rather than being a failure, recognize that everyone is perfectly entitled to miss a work out every so often or have an off-day regarding eating healthily.

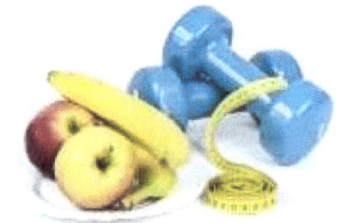

Don't let it knock your confidence.
One day won't prevent you from reaching your goals. Put things in perspective. A missed workout or slip up doesn't undo all of the hard work you had accomplished. and it doesn't mean you have to start all over again. Think about it as a day trip - time off for good behavior - then pick up where you left off and continue with all your good actions.

Make simple changes, add to them gradually and you WILL lose weight.

Use Your Social Network

Post it, Tweet it, Blog it. Use your social network to receive words of encouragement and support.

Everyone needs to hear a few words of support and encouragement every now and again, and there is no better place to go than to the people who love you and a family that was glad to see you healthier and happier, so don't underestimate their support.

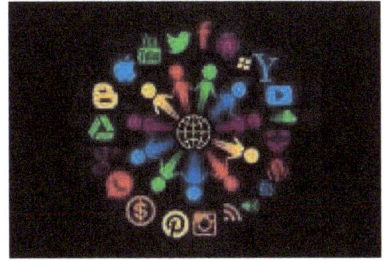

So if you are striving towards a major goal post it, tweet it, blog it. Put it out there. Once you have made your goals public it keeps you accountable, makes taking steps to success far less daunting and overwhelming and you can be up built by messages of support and encouragement.

Not only that, but by sharing your goals online you may find that one of your friends in your social network is aiming for the same goals and can add to your support system. How great would that be?

Make Simple Changes and Add to Them Gradually

We said earlier that to be successful, you need to take lots of smaller steps not huge ones and this applies within the areas we need to make changes in. Trying to change all your eating habits overnight can prove to be a massive challenge. one that could derail your efforts to change. It is much better and far less stressful to adopt just one or two healthy habit changes at a time, rather than overwhelm yourself with a huge list of them. Small, simple changes will help you reach your goals far easier than a dramatic lifestyle overhaul all at the same time.

Decide to do one or two small things each day or week, such as reducing the portions of your food or carrying a water bottle with you to keep you hydrated during the day.

Once those little changes have become part of your routine, move on and add another couple of changes and so on. Taking these smaller steps will help you accept and get used to each change. which means you become more able to stick with each new change rather than allowing them overwhelming you into giving up.

Don't Be Negative

Instead of starving yourself, starve the negative thoughts that say: You CANT lose weight in a healthy way, and feed the POSITIVE thoughts that say: **YOU CAN.** Determination. Motivation. I will: I can: I have; I want to.

All these thoughts express positivity to succeed, and having a positive attitude is the way you need to train your mind to think. It's not always easy to avoid the negative thoughts that will make you want to give up your goals. It's easier to convince yourself that you are never going to lose the weight, especially if you are not seeing the results a coming as fast as you would like them.

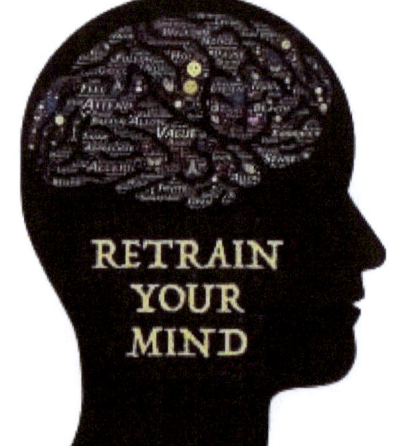

Remember that every little bit of progress that you make, no matter how small, is still progress! Even if you only lose half a pound a week, in a year that is 26Ib - almost 2 stone or 12 kg! How could that ever be anything other than a huge positive?

Stay Away from Bad Influences

We all have them - weaknesses that speak to the rebellious inner self and that we give in to without much of a struggle. Sometimes, they can sneak up on us when we are unprepared, like the fast food restaurants that are on every street corner when we are hungry.

Other times, they are places we have to go past like certain supermarket aisle or the bakery shop window. It could even be that well intentioned friends try to tempt you into making a 'just this once' unhealthy choice. As hard as it may be in the beginning, you need to try to avoid these triggers as they can lead you to start back on those unhealthy

Keep a Success Journal

When faced with the challenge of losing weight, our mind can quickly forget all of the victories we have achieved and blow all the bad things out of proportion, but if you keep a record of them yourself, then this discouraging tendency can be overcome.

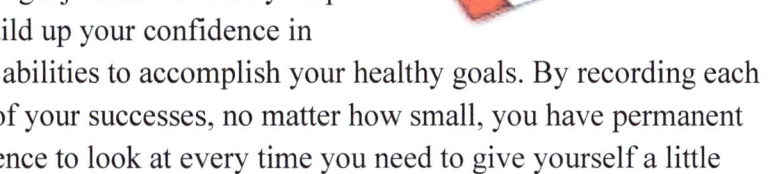

Writing a journal can really help to build up your confidence in your abilities to accomplish your healthy goals. By recording each one of your successes, no matter how small, you have permanent evidence to look at every time you need to give yourself a little encouragement or motivation to keep going.

If you have a smartphone there are many fitness and journal apps, which can help you keep a success journal. Not only will you be able to carry your journal around with you but it will be instantly at your fingertips whenever you need to make an entry or remind yourself how well you are doing.

Write Down One Reason Why Losing Weight is Bad for You

Unless you are at the right weight now, you want to lose weight because you know you aren't as healthy as you could be. Make a list of as many reasons as you can why losing weight is bad for you. Can you think of any?

Now write down all of the reasons you can think about why losing weight is good for you. You should be looking at all the ways to reinforce the message within yourself that losing weight is a GOOD thing, so by making sure your list is a nice long positive list, you reinforce the motivation to lose weight and stick to your plans.

- Fewer Employment Opportunities
- High Blood Pressure
- Type 2 Diabetes
- Bone Problems
- Hernia
- Arthritis
- Limited Mobility
- Increased Sweating
- Social Discrimination
- Breathing Problems
- High Cholesterol
- Joint Problems
- Cancer
- Low Self-Esteem
- Heart Attack
- Depression
- Deep Vein Thrombosis
- Lower Life Expectancy

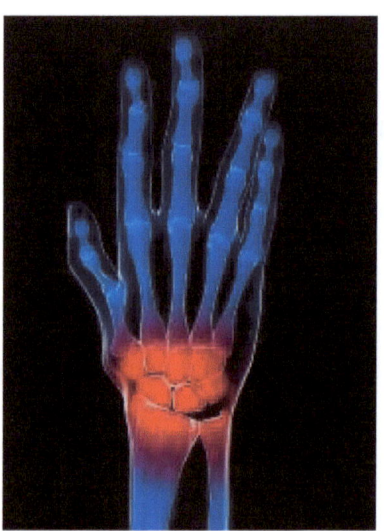

Know Yourself

Understand who you are as an individual. This will let you see why you make the choices you do, which is so important in keeping you motivated.

So instead of working against your natural tendencies, work with them. For example, if you are a walker don't try to force yourself into becoming a marathon runner. If you enjoy the company of others and are naturally sociable then take a fitness class with a friend or join a group.

Keep It Simple

There is really no such thing as a quick fix. Quick fix routes, such as sweat suits or extreme diets, don't work for the majority of people because they hold out an unrealistic end result. Unless you only have 5-10 pounds to lose, these ways to weight loss can do your personal self-esteem more damage that the weight you are carrying and so you should avoid them at all costs.

Instead, keep things simple. Slowly and gradually reach your goals without taking extreme measures that only have temporary, if any, effect. Some examples of keeping things simple and making small changes would be by adding sparking water to your usual orange juice at breakfast, or making your sandwich with one less slice of bread and adding lettuce instead. You will be able to think of many other things where making very small changes can produce major, lasting effects and give you great results.

Donate Your Fat Clothes

If you choose to hold on to your heavier clothes just in case you don't lose the weight or worse, regain what you have lost, you have immediately set yourself up to fail.

You are telling yourself that you have no confidence at all that you will be able to succeed. In which case, it is very probable that you will give up very quickly.

Put your money where your mouth is: donate them to your favorite charity and then move on. By getting rid of the clothes that no longer fit you and visualizing yourself in a new wardrobe. you can picture how great your body feels and the thrill of wearing all those new clothes, getting rid of the possibility that you will go back to your unhealthy habits.

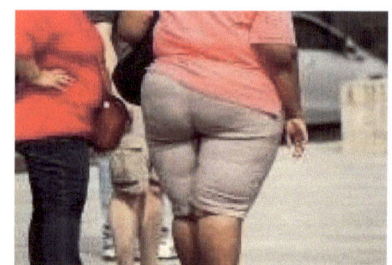

Staying positive will help you stay motivated. Small steps will eventually see you right at the top of any mountain you choose to climb, with a successful healthier you at the end of it all.

You can take this one step further by photographing your progress every few months. Nothing makes more impression on showing you how far you have come and on your self-esteem than to see the way your body is changing shape for the better as you progress.

Your journal and photographic record are very personal things, so you may feel better keeping these to yourself. If so, then by password protecting your app or computer folder, or hiding your journal in a safe place, it will allow you to write down all of your private thoughts and keep them away from prying eyes.

Try and find people, places and things that you find inspirational and will have a more positive influence on your lifestyle. Keep yourself busy and positive and this will help you to reach your goals.

The key to losing weight and keeping it off is balance and a positive attitude. This will motivate you to keep on losing weight.

Conclusion

With the right planning and goal setting, any major project is achievable. Weight loss is no different! Nothing will make weight loss easy. but the right advice can be all you need to kick start your weight loss program into high gear! Read on for valuable information to help you attain your goals in weight loss and keep you on that healthier path.

A good way to lose weight is to reduce the amount of time you rest between sets when you are lifting weights. By reducing the amount of time you rest between sets, you burn more calories and in a way, you're combining cardio and weights into one workout session.

Never let yourself get too hungry. Keep a small container of fresh, raw vegetables, plain raw almonds or cut-up fruit to munch on whenever you start to get hungry. Small, healthy snacks throughout the day keep your energy up and help you resist the temptation to go crazy with high-calorie food.

When attempting to lose weight, be sure that you do not fall victim to the purging of recently eaten food. If this does occur, it is a sickness and you should consult with a doctor or counselor for guidance. Not only is your body not getting the nutrients that it needs, you are harming your esophagus and teeth as well.

Use inspirational quotes to help you in your weight loss journey. When you are in the throes of a powerful food craving, it is sometimes difficult to remember the commitment you have made to good health.

Try putting quotes on your refrigerator, inside your pantry doors and other places you will notice them, to help you stop for a second and get refocused on your goal.

Visualization can be an important tool for weight loss. When you are craving an unhealthy food, or just feel like snacking, close your eyes and imagine the way you looked when you were at your ideal weight. This process helps you remember why you want to lose the weight in the first place.

Substituting low fat processed foods for high fat ones when trying to lose weight is a very popular idea; however, it does not always work. For example, replacing regular store bought muffins with low fat store bought muffins may make you want to eat two of the low fat muffins instead of one! The low fat ones are usually missing some of the taste of the regular muffins. Instead, try making your own muffins and other food! You will know what is going into what you are making and can cut back on certain things without sacrificing taste.

One way to encourage yourself to lose weight is to keep a pair of cute jeans that are just a little too small in your closet. They don't even have to be one size too small, just a little too snug to be able to wear out of the house. Try them on at least once a week. You will be happy when your diligence pays off because you will look smokin' in your "new" old jeans.

Short of hiring a personal trainer, most of us are on our own when it comes to weight loss. We need to be informed and stay motivated. Know what works and stick with it! Take what you have learned from this article and use it as a guide to lose weight and become a stronger, healthier and happier individual!

Other Health Reports by This Author

If you would like to read more health reports on various topics, here is a list of CreateSpace titles and descriptions:

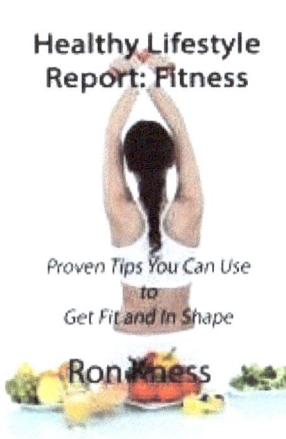

Fitness

So how much will you need to work out to feel these benefits of exercising? That all depends on your current fitness levels. The good news is that just 30 minutes of exercise a day is enough to improve your health drastically. So what are you waiting for! Let's dig deeper into the world of fitness and how it can improve your life now and into the future.

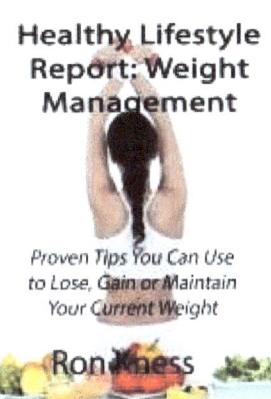

Weight Management

Losing weight in theory is easy. All you have to do is burn more calories than what you eat. If your deficit is 3,500 calories in a week, you'll lose one pound.

The problem is there are many more factors at play that can affect weight loss than just calories, such as emotions, stress, illness, hormones, menstruation, etc. So it is not easy, but with a healthy lifestyle program it is doable.

Nutrition

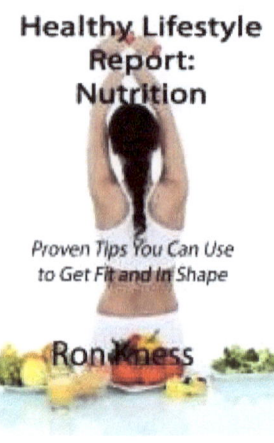

Nutrition is at the heart of losing weight and good health. In fact 80% of weight loss has to do with eating healthy with the other 20% about exercise. Good nutrition starts with three areas:

- What you eat

- How much you eat

- When you eat.

Senior Health

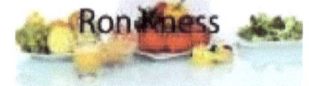

Retirement should be one of the best times of your life, but health issues caused by being overweight can not only limit your mobility, but cause a whole host of health problems. In this report, we discuss how to eat right, exercise and deal with some of the issues of aging.

Be sure to check back at CreateSpace at *https://www.createspace.com* frequently for new health reports. Just go to the Store and Search for "Ron Kness" (without the quotes of course) for a list of my books and reports.

About the Author

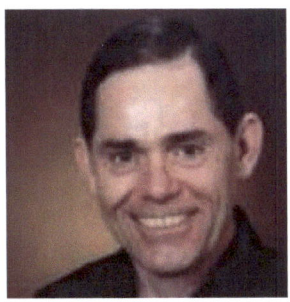 I grew up in Central Minnesota, where my parents owned and operated a fishing resort. Once out of high school I tried a couple of semesters of college, only to quit halfway through the Spring term; I decided at that time that college wasn't for me.

Then I decided to follow my father's previous occupation as an auto mechanic. I graduated from a two-year of vocational training course and worked as a mechanic. While in vocational training, I decided to join the National Guard where I eventually ended up working full-time for 32 years.

So how does all of this relate to writing? In one of my leadership schools, the instructor, who was an English teacher at a juvenile detention center, presented writing to me in a whole new way - a way that started to develop my interest in working with words.

Fast forward about 40 years and I now have over 50 books listed on Amazon for Kindle and CreateSpace.

Besides my own writing, I also ghostwrite ebooks, reports, articles, blogs and do Kindle conversions for my clients on a variety of topics.

Today my wife and I live in Gold Canyon, AZ, where you'll find me happily sitting in my office typing away on my laptop as I work on my next book or ghostwriting project . . . that is if we are not traveling on a cruise ship - our new-found mode of travel.

www.ingramcontent.com/pod-product-compliance
Lightning Source LLC
Chambersburg PA
CBHW050859290526
45792CB00002B/653